Edward S. Steven

The best preliminary education for the study of medicine

Edward S. Stevens

The best preliminary education for the study of medicine

ISBN/EAN: 9783742822864

Manufactured in Europe, USA, Canada, Australia, Japa

Cover: Foto ©Lupo / pixelio.de

Manufactured and distributed by brebook publishing software
(www.brebook.com)

Edward S. Stevens

The best preliminary education for the study of medicine

By EDWARD S. STEV...

A wise physician, skill'd our wounds
Is more than armies to the common

LEBANON, O.:
THE WESTERN STAR PRINT.

By an order adopted in 1826, the Secretary was directed to publish annually the following votes:

1st. That the Board do not consider themselves as approving the doctrines contained in any of the dissertations to which premiums are adjudged,

2d. That in case of publication of a successful dissertation, the author be considered as bound to print the above vote in connection therewith.

THE BEST PRELIMINARY EDUCATION FOR THE STUDY OF MEDICINE.

PART I.

REQUIRED PRELIMINARY WORK.

This essay will be written from an American stand-point, and will be divided into three parts. Part I will speak of the required preliminary work for the study of medicine; Part II will speak of what constitutes a preliminary medical education, and of the manner in which a person intending to study medicine should conduct his educational course; Part III will offer a model for a college course of study.

That the medical profession is becoming awake to its interests in the subject of medical education and medical requirements is evidenced by the following facts: 1. In 1876 a convention of medical colleges assembled in Philadelphia, "To consider all matters relating to reform in medical college work." This resulted in the formation of the American Medical College Association, the object of

which was to be "the advancement of medical education."
2. Many of the best medical colleges have within recent
years been announcing in their annual circulars a matriculation examination.   3. The recently delivered Presidential
addresses of a number of State Medical Societies have
considered particularly the subject of medical education.
4. At the meeting of the American Medical Association
of 1884 an amendment to the Constitution was offered of
which the following is a portion: "No person who shall
hereafter graduate from a medical college where literary
education is not a prerequisite to such graduation, shall be
eligible to be a delegate to the American Medical Association." 5. The American Academy of Medicine, an association organized less than a dozen years ago, requires of
candidates for membership the possession of a literary
degree.   6. Several State Boards of Health refuse longer
to recognize the diplomas of such medical schools as do not
require of their matriculants some evidence of preliminary
training.

So then there is an evident consent in the profession
as to what ought to be done for its elevation, but there is
a general backwardness about initiating a forward march.
There is a selfish vein in our natures which forbids our
acting independently for the good of medical science.

What requirements are made by American medical
colleges in the way of preliminary training? By the
majority of colleges no requirement is made at all.   By
those colleges which demand the passing of a preliminary
examination, for the most part the requirements are not
of a high order.   If the student be a graduate of a literary

college, a high school, or an academy ; if he has already passed the entrance examination in a literary, or medical college ; if he has a county or state teacher's certificate ; if he is a graduate in medicine of some other college ; or if he is a special student, not working for a degree,—the examination is not required. If he cannot give any such evidence of his fitness to pursue the study of medicine he must pass an examination "in the branches of a good English education."

A good English education is variously understood. By most of the colleges there is no further expression of the requirements than is given in the sentence above. One college specifies the examination to be in "English Grammar, History, Geography, Arithmetic, Elementary Physics, and Composition."

The following is the examination offered by the Woman's Medical College of the New York Infirmary :

1. Orthography, English Composition, and Penmanship, by means of a page written at the·time and place of examination.

2. Definitions and Synonyms as found in "The Scholar's Companion."

3. Latin, through Declensions and Conjugations.

4. Arithmetic, in Denominate Numbers, Fractions, Proportions, Percentage, and the Roots.

5. Algebra—Davies' Elementary,—through simple equations.

6. Geometry—Davies' Legendre,— first and second books.

7. Botany, Physics, and Chemistry, as found in

"Science Primers," edited by Profs. Huxley, Roscoe, and Balfour Stewart.

The Medical School of Harvard University requires in Latin "the translation of easy prose." The candidate is required to pass an approved examination in any one of the following branches: French, German, the Elements of Algebra or Plane Geometry, Botany. These are in addition to the usual examinations in English and Physics. First year students who satisfy the Faculty that they have already had a sufficient training in General Chemistry are permitted to pass over this branch, and may proceed at once to the study of Medical Chemistry.

At the University of Michigan the candidate "will be asked to give an account of his previous educational advantages, and to answer such questions in arithmetic, geography, and history, and on forms of government and current events, as shall show his general intelligence; and particularly will he be required to correct imperfect English and to show his ability to express ideas correctly in writing. Since many present themselves a long time after completing their school education, the examination will not be technical, nor in the rules of school books. The aim will be to ascertain the results of the candidate's previous training, and his present practical capacity and ability to appreciate the technical study of medicine."

It will be seen that a high grade of scholarship is not demanded. The examinations except at a few colleges are such as most boys of fourteen should be able to pass.

Some of the colleges make no requirements for entrance because "students are *presumed* to have the necessary education for undertaking the study of medicine." A few colleges offer an optional examination in order that their graduates may be spared the trouble of passing an examination before certain State Boards.

A very fair examination is offered to persons desirous of entering the Medical Corps of the U. S. Army. The following general plan of the examination (so far as it refers to preliminary training) is taken from the U. S. Army Regulations:

I. A short essay, either autobiographical or upon some professional subject—to be indicated by the Board.

II. Physical examination. This will be rigid, and each candidate will in addition, be required to certify " *that he labors under no mental or physical infirmity, nor disability of any kind, which can in any way interfere with the most efficient discharge of any duty which may be required.*"

III. Oral examinations on subjects of preliminary education, general literature and general science. The Board will satisfy itself by an actual examination that the candidate possesses a thorough knowledge of the branches taught in the common schools, especially of *English Grammar, Arithmetic, and History and Geography of the United States.* Any candidate *found deficient in these branches will not be examined further.*

Oral examination on general science will include Chemistry and Natural Philosophy; and that on general literature will embrace English literature, Latin and general History, ancient and modern. Candidates claiming proficiency in other branches of knowledge such as the higher mathematics, the ancient and modern languages, etc., will be examined therein, and receive due credit therefor. This gives a general idea of the preliminary training that is considered necessary in the United States. The U. S. Army requirements hint at the desirability of a higher education. The traditions of a country influence its customs in a great degree. It is in part on account of traditions that American requirements are so low, and that those of certain European countries are as high as they are. This may be shown by a reference to the requirements in Canada, our near neighbor. The College of Physicians and Surgeons of the Province of Quebec offer the following matriculation examination:

Compulsory Subjects:—English, French, Latin, Arithmetic, Algebra, Euclid, History, Geography, Belles-Lettres.

Optional Subjects:—Candidates can select any one of the following: Greek, Natural and Moral Philosophy.

The examinations in Canada are similar to those in England, whence many of her traditions came, and presume a higher grade of scholarship than the examinations in the United States.

For the purpose of comparison and perhaps of obtaining some useful suggestion it may be well to take a glance at the preliminary requirements in the mother country. In the first place although the possession of a degree in arts exempts one from the preliminary examination the Universities whose diplomas are accepted are particularly mentioned. The Royal College of Surgeons of England, offers an examination which may be taken as a type of the English tests of preliminary training. The following is taken from the "regulations respecting the education and examination of Candidates for the Diploma of Member" of the Royal College of Surgeons.

PART I.

Compulsory Subjects.

1. Writing from Dictation.
2. English Grammar.
3. Writing a short English composition; such as a description of a place, an account of some useful or natural product, or the like.
4. Arithmetic. No candidate will be passed who does not show a competent knowledge of the first four rules, simple and compound, of Vulgar Fractions, and of Decimals.
5. Questions on the Geography of Europe, and particularly of the British Isles.
6. Questions on the outlines of English History, that is, the succession of the Soverigns and the leading events of each reign.
7. Mathematics. Euclid, Books I. and II., or the subjects thereof; Algebra to Simple Equations inclusive.
8. Translation of a passage from the second book of Cæsar's Commentaries "De Bello Gallico."

PART II.

Optional Subjects.

Papers will also be set on the following seven subjects and each Candidate will be required to offer himself for examination on one subject at least, at his option, but no

Candidate will be allowed to offer himself for examination on more than four subjects:—

1. Translation of a passage from the first Book of the Anabasis of Xenophon.

2. Translation of a passage from X. B. Saintines's "Picciola."

3. Translation of a passage from Schiller's "Wilhelm Tell."

Besides these Translations into English, the Candidate will be required to answer questions on the Grammar of each subject, whether compulsory or optional.

4. Mechanics. The question will be chiefly of an elementary character.

5. Chemistry. The questions will be on the elementary facts of Chemistry.

6. Botany and Zoology. The questions will be on the classification of Plants and Animals.

7. Euclid, Books, III., IV., V. and VI.

The quality of the handwriting and the spelling will be taken into account.

Note.—A Candidate in order to qualify for the Membership is required to pass at one and the same Examination, in all the subjects of Part I and in one subject of Part II, and failure in any one of those subjects necessitates re-examination in all. A Candidate in order to qualify for the Fellowship is required, in addition to the subjects of Part I, to pass in not less than four, at his option, of the subjects in Part II.

In Germany the preliminary training is of longer duration and is more extensive than in England or America. The license to practice medicine is granted by the State. To obtain a degree and license to practice the student must first of all be a graduate of a gymnasium or other school equal to a gymnasium in thoroughness and standing. Men of defective preparation may pursue the course under certain circumstances and may receive a certificate stating that they have pursued given studies, and such men may keep a drug-store, but cannot practice medicine. The gymnasim course covers a period of nine years. There are six working days to the week, and eight or nine hours to the day of schoolwork. There are two half holidays allowed each week, and only ten weeks of vacation divided through the year. The drill in Latin and Greek is long and thorough. The whole course is steady hard work.

In America the preliminary requirements are by no means exclusive. Any one at all capable of attending the sick can make his entrance to a college of medicine. But the question that we wish to consider is not of *necessary* preliminary education, but of the *best* preliminary education for the study of medicine. Any one whose aspirations are high must be, in a measure, an independent worker. A good student will work beyond what is absolutely required. Literary schools have seen this and have thrown out the very tempting bait of preparatory departments in medicine. The John Hopkins University in its presenta·tion of various courses of study has arranged a group preliminary to medical studies. "Opportunities are here afforded to a young man," says University Circular No. 23, "who expects at a later day to take up the study of medicine, to become proficient in laboratory work while acquiring a knowledge of German and French, and continuing his general education." The Medical Faculty of Harvard University, too, advise "those who intend to study Medicine to pay special attention to the study of Natural History, Chemistry, Physics, and the French and German languages, while in college."

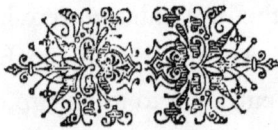

PART II.

THE BEST PRELIMINARY EDUCATION FOR THE STUDY OF MEDICINE.

In the regulations of the U. S. Army Medical Department are found the requirements of soundness as to "morals, habits, physical and mental qualifications, and general aptitude for the service." It would be well if they were made requirements by the student himself for entering the army of world workers. In part they will be spoken of in this portion of the essay.

In the consideration of the "best preliminary education for the study of medicine" one of the first thoughts that presents itself is that the student should prepare himself for the hard work which he is sure to find in the honest study and practice of medicine by not only building up a strong constitution, but also by learning how to care for the temple in which his mind is to dwell. As medical training is conducted at present in the United States a good *physique*

is necessary to successfully undergo it. More than that,—
without robust health the student may even fail in the
midst of his preliminary work. There are too many boys
who find out too late that all of education is not to be
found locked up in books. And so I would have the
student learn first of all how to divide his time between
mental occupation, physical exercise, and the lighter
forms of recreation. The story of Mr. Blaikie is to be
listened to with something more than the interest one
might put in a simple narrative of fact. There is in it a
lesson that we may all well heed.

In the pursuance of the physical education compan-
ionship is desirable. "Athletics are essentially a popular
pursuit, conducive to good citizenship, and the cultivation
of which, therefore, good citizenship should imply. * *
* * There is rivalry in athletics, of course, but much
less of petty jealousy than an outsider would suppose;
not nearly so much, for example, as subsists between
eminent astronomers in search of a comet, or fashionable
ladies in search of a new sensation. " (*Julian Hawthorne*).
This very rivalry is one of the pleasant and profitable
features of the "building of the muscle." When brothers
or friends interest themselves in the same form of bodily
exercise and practice it together, the mental relaxation is
more complete than when practiced in solitude, and the
glow of health is brighter and comes sooner. But this is
to be kept in mind—quoting from the same essay—"health
is, or should be, incidental to this pleasure; that is to say,
I question the propriety of making health the deliberate
object of exercise. Let it come if it will; but it will come

none the slower if you forbear to be on the watch for it."

How shall physical development be best promoted? With all boys sports, especially out-of-door sports, should be encouraged. A boy should not live many years before learning to swim, skate, and ride. There are a great many boys who do not learn either of these at an early age unless it be the second. There are few sports that are more pleasurable, and are there any that will contribute more to muscular development? To these I would add, as particularly to be encouraged, boating, and the use of boxing gloves. Walking as a sport is too much neglected, while running as a part of some modern games is sometimes overdone.

I have spoken of sports for boys and the question is of the preparation of men. The perfect man is but the perfect boy grown up. There are some points in this discussion that are general. It is not necessary to make a special point in development for the production of a physician or surgeon. If the man is built symmetrically in mind and body, he is ready for almost any pursuit. There are some exercises which are useful for the development of particular faculties, and which might be classed under the head of physical exercises. Among these might be mentioned rifle practice, which requires an accurate eye and a steady hand. Did not our professor of operative surgery mention these same qualifications as essential for the successful surgeon?

There is a method of promoting muscular growth that is particularly useful for students, and one that can be pursued daily during one's whole life. I refer to the exercises of the gymnasium. , With many young men the using of dumb-bells and Indian clubs is a favorite way of affording mental relaxation and muscular tonicity. William Cullen Bryant was in the habit of using dumb-bells for half an hour or more each morning, and of walking to his office, and he thought that his health and strength were preserved by this habit. Perhaps his idea was true only in part. One of the advantages of dumb-bells and clubs is that they can be used within doors, and by persons whose time is limited.

There are many persons who will neglect an exercise which has no other object than simple muscular development. They can derive no pleasure from the use of dumb-bells, clubs, or weights; bar or trapeze; perhaps they do not enjoy the common sports of boys and young men,— and all because they can see no good end in them. Such a person might employ himself regurlarly in the performance of certain necessary tasks, such as, for instance, the regular care of a horse. The work that is required for the attention that a horse ought to have will in a few weeks make a perceptible change in the shape of a weakly young man's chest, and will cause his pectorals and bicipitals to become larger and firmer. His step will become lighter, and his carriage more erect.

It is not only brute strength that a young man should endeavor to attain. There is a delicacy of touch and a certain sleight in the performance of one's duties that is worth striving for. The education of the sense of touch is one of the things medical students are admonished to attend to. It comes to some men more readily than to others, and to those soonest, I believe, who are accustomed to exercises requiring skill. There are some of the mechanical arts that will assist in the development of this faculty, among which might be mentioned the art of turning in wood and metal. There are other advantages in the cultivation of this art which might be alluded to. The use of tools is acquired. Has not every physician felt the need of this accomplishment? I have heard instrument makers speak rather slightingly of medical men because "they were not mechanics." If one will but look at the clumsily contrived instruments that are every day being invented by medical men a reason for the remark will be seen. The inventive faculty is stimulated by this work. It is very convenient for the young surgeon to be able to fit his own appliances. Frequently it is necessary for him to do it with few materials at his command. Is not this sufficient reason for the prospective medical student to engage in this or a similar employment?

This is an age when women fit themselves for entrance into the ranks of the medical profession. For them in this connection I cannot do better than to quote from Emmet: "If on account of fitness of mental capacity and force of circumstances, it is deemed advisable that a young woman should acquire the higher branches of education, she should not attempt it without having gained the most perfect physical development. She should spend the same years in the completion of her education that are given by the young man to his collegiate course, for she will then have reached a more suitable age and will be in better physical condition for the acquisition of knowledge." In the preceding paragraphs,

written as though to young men, little has been said that
might not be as well applied to young women.

Another part of education, not often enough considered, relates to morals. No matter how much reverence
may be paid the *physician*, the *medical student* has been, is
now, almost in a condition of ostracism, and strange as it
may seem many of them do not care, or perhaps even take
a reckless delight in it. The bad practices of medical students of earlier days are copied too closely to-day. Are
the colleges careful enough in examining the '' proper tes-
timonials of character'' which they demand? At least a
late author says, ''we have many wolves in sheep's clothing
among us. If the testimony of the sufferers is to be
accepted, it is evident that we have more abortionists in
the profession than out of it.'' I do not wish to speak too
harshly of the medical profession. I would but call attention to the necessity of greater care in this matter.

Let those who look to medicine as their field of work
learn to look upon the noble art as something more than a
means of livelihood. Let the young man learn that unless
he can bring with him a great deal of sympathy for hu-
manity he is not ''called'' to the ranks of medicine.
'' How much the family physician can do to set lives right
morally as well as physically, to allay social discord, to
correct misunderstandings, to comfort the sorrowing, to
give garments of praise for the spirit of heaviness, to rouse
a slumbering will, sometimes to reclaim the profligate,
enforcing the highest lessons of virtue from the penalties
of disease, in short to make men, women and children
healthier, happier, better.'' (*Parvin.*) Perhaps it is not

the whole of life to live; there may be in it a cold side
dish to serve as food for the medical scientist;—and yet
the *living* does constitute the important part of life, and
the living beings are continually crying for help in the
midst of their physical, mental, and moral infirmities, and
the physician is often the only one who can answer their
prayers.

Before discussing the question of mental training,
there is a subject which ought to be spoken of, and which
if heeded would save a vast amount of unnecessary expen-
diture of nerve force.   Hurry and worry are the peculiar
faults of the American people.   The student should early
learn that there is sufficient time for his work, if he does
not waste it.   There is no great problem waiting to be
solved by him, that cannot wait until his period of careful
preparation is at an end.   If he is capable, he will do better work if he does not begin his professional career too·
early.   The finest and largest crystals are formed very
slowly.   That the preliminary work of a medical student
may be thorough it is necessary that he give considerable
time to it.   Too many do their work in race-horse style,—
they try to make the fastest possible time with the lightest
possible weight.

In considering the question of preliminary medical
education it is to be borne in mind that the cabalistic letters
of a degree, and the social influence that the college graduate might possibly have, are not the things sought for.
This view is seen by the eyes of the charlatan only..   The
student may be one of rare abilities, an average man, or as
is frequently the case, one of an inferior grade of intellect.

The same course and arrangement of study will not fit the mind and convenience of every individual; or given the same course, the brighter mind will accomplish the work sooner and better. This question involves not only a *what* but a *how* as well.

An education—using the term in its most common sense—may be obtained in or out of a school. Which is the better way? A person's circumstances may demand the latter. If it can be done the young man will get his best education at a school. "The proper study of mankind is man," and the life of a physician is a continued study of mankind. The best preparation for a life among men is a life among boys and younger men. If a boy's first knowledge of books is obtained in a class with other boys, he gets at the same time his first lesson in a study apart from books, which may be fully as valuable to him as the a, b, c. He will learn to see failures and successes; little strifes and jealousies; the noble action of one as against the littleness of another. Is not this the picture of a little world? In this is one of the great advantages of the common school system. The student learns to know his fellows.

A word about books. A knowledge of how to make a proper use of books determines the successful student. The student should learn to study the subject he is working upon, and not merely the ideas of some one book. He should learn that possibly there is more of value on his subject out of books than in. In many cases the work that is done with books is supplemental to work of another kind. For instance when instruction is given by lectures

the careful student, either with or without notes, will con-
sult not one but all works to which he may have access,
which may afford any fresh light on the subject before him.
Again, in laboratory work his books give the student di-
rections for work, and indicate the work and the particulars
of the work that has already been done, but his own ob-
servations and his verification of the work of others is of
far more value than anything he can read. Another use
of books is for recitations. In the most common method
of doing recitation work the members of the class all use
the same book, the instructor gives a certain number of
pages to the class for a lesson, and at the appointed hour
he hears the lesson recited, often requiring the language of
the book. This method is necessary for younger students,
and is well enough in certain studies where the memory is
being trained. With older students the method can be
improved upon, particularly in the purely scientific studies.
A newer, livelier interest would be excited if the instructor
would indicate a subject for study and the range that would
be allowed for the class work, and then leave the student
to work in his own way. Assistance might be given the
class by a list of authorities to be consulted. In a certain
post-graduate course one of the professors will lecture
upon a subject in which he has had special experience, and
at the same time he will have before the class upon the
black-board the bibliography of the subject.

I have indicated most of the methods of study usually
pursued in the schools—by lectures, by laboratory work,
and by recitations. Each has its mission to fulfill. In
many schools too many lectures are given, for many a lec-

turer having no originality about him simply gives a re-hash of what he finds in the books. The lecture is a relic of the first days of the university. To-day it is only needed where original unpublished work has been done, or where the lecturer has had some special advantages for observation, or some experience of an unusual kind. Occasionally a school has in its faculty men with an individuality that is manifested in no way so well as in their speaking. Their very presence is a stimulus to the student to good work. For such men the lecture room is the proper place. In some of the scientific studies a valuable working method is the study of nature face to face. There is much of interest in this method of work, and for some parts of life study it is the only true way. It offers a change from indoor work and promotes the well-being of the physical man. An exercise to which not enough attention is paid is the doing of original work. A little of this might be done in almost every department of school work.

When we prepare to build we lay a foundation that will support whatever superstructure we propose to erect. In the preparation for a work of study the same principle should be observed, and a broad, deep, and firm foundation should be laid. Studies are disciplinary and semi-professional. The former class should take precedence. Sometimes the practical studies can be used so as to afford excellent mental discipline. But the student should remember that during his course of study he is only laying his foundation, and the only reference he should have to the superstructure is to see that the foundation is in harmony with the work that is to crown it.

There has been almost a war between the scientists and the progressive, practical men on one side, and on the other those who would still adhere to the classics and mathematics as chief among the studies which are to mold the student's mind. It is hardly within the province of this essay to treat of the subject generally, but as far as it relates to the "best preliminary education for the study of medicine" it becomes necessary to speak of the two old languages, Latin and Greek, and their old-time comrade Mathematics. *Festina lente*, says the old proverb. Perhaps we are making too rapid a change from the old traditional course of study to the more modern one of the practical men.

Shall the prospective medical student study the Latin and Greek languages?—is a question often debated, and one that is not always satisfactorily answered. Many students feel that their time is limited, and that they must hurry to and through their medical studies for the sake of bread and raiment. If such a person will study medicine it makes little difference whether he makes any study of these languages or not. Perhaps it would be better for him not to get a simple smattering of them. But even he might get a sufficient knowledge of "prescription Latin" to prevent his ending a prescription

R. Aquæ q. s. . . . . add . . . 8 ounces, which is not only barbarous Latin, but also a curious mixture of two languages; nevertheless the expression was used in a recent medical journal just as I have given it. But we started out with the proposition that the student was to have the *best* education and that he should give sufficient time to it. In that case he should give several years of his time to daily work on Latin and Greek. The first reason for this is that the languages afford an excellent means of mental discipline. It is claimed by the progressive men that the modern languages are fully equivalent to the older languages for this purpose, and that they have the additional advantage of being useful, being living. If we are to insist upon the combination of the useful with the disciplinary we may still hold to our classics. An example has been given above of the result of the "little Latin and less Greek" sort of education in faulty prescription writing. There is perhaps no profession, besides that of medicine, that to so great a degree takes its scientific terms—their name is Legion, and they are of frequent coinage—from the Latin and Greek. To be sure the student could look out the derivation of his words in Webster or Dunglison, but he is best equipped who can read them as he runs. But this is not the end. The Latin language especially lends color to the thoughts of working scholars. Is it best that the student be born from the matrix of preparatory life to the world of active life color-blind?

Mention has been made of the modern languages, meaning by them the German and French, and perhaps we might also include the Italian. Probably they have a value fully equal to the older languages as means of discipline if they are properly utilized, but as they are frequently studied they are no more useful than Latin and Greek—probably not as much so. To do the student any practical good they must be so thoroughly learned that he shall be able to at least read them readily, and it would be that much better if he was sufficiently familiar with them to converse in them. The reason for this thorough knowledge of these languages is found in the special uses to which the student may apply them. The chief advantage of a knowledge of German and French is that through them fresh resources in the shape of foreign books and journals are opened to the student for reference in his work. Ability to read easily is necessary for this purpose. Another advantage is to the student who expects to gain a portion of his medical education in foreign countries. Still a third advantage of a knowledge of these languages lies in the fact that after student life the physician can make use of his acquisition in communicating with those of his patients who speak only those languages. This use is, so far as the subject of this essay is concerned, a minor one, but for this purpose and for foreign study the knowledge of the languages must be such that the student may speak, and understand when others speak. In order to gain this thorough familiarity with these languages the best plan is to begin their study early in life. It may be well done in one of two ways. One is by living in a family where no other language is spoken except the one the student wishes to acquire. The other is by school work. In some public schools German is taught in the lowest grades. In most private schools the younger scholars may study French, and in some they may study Italian. It is not always convenient for the student to make a careful study of each of these languages. In case a part only are studied I would put them down as to their value in the order that they have already been mentioned—German, French, Italian.

Of mathematics little need be said, as it bears but little closer relationship to the study of medicine than it does to almost every trade and profession. Elementary mathematics is necessary to civilized life. Higher mathematics may not be absolutely necessary to the successful student and physician, but he who has given his time and attention to these studies is better prepared for work than the one who has not.

There are a thousand and one ways in which mathematics comes to the student's assistance. The chief value of the study to the medical man is for its training. It exercises the reason and judgment in a manner as no other work will do. Do you ask why so many and such various studies are advised, which have for their main object simply mental exercise? The answer might be given that it is for a reason similiar to that which advises so many and such various exercises for the development of the muscular system. As one set of exercises brings into play first this group of muscles and then that; so the other set calls into action now one of the faculties of the mind, and now another. There is one branch of mathematics in which the student of natural science has a special interest—the mathematics of physics, chemistry, and astronomy; and according as the student, whose aim is medicine, wishes to be thoroughly prepared every way he will consider the importance of mathematics, and its relation to the natural sciences.

The student should remember that there are other

things to be thought of than those which seemingly have a direct bearing upon his future calling. The physician as much as any man should be prepared to look out upon his fellows, and to mingle with them in general social meetings. He as much as another should be able not only to give advice on general sanitary matters, but as well to discuss the rights and wrongs of state polity.

The next group of studies to be considered have for their object the drawing of the attention. of the student to the ways and doings of people. It includes history and literature. These studies have also the object of imparting a general culture which the student should cultivate. The physician may also be a gentleman.

There is no one who should not have a good knowledge of the history of his own country. The very careful student will do more than this. Realizing the advantage of a knowledge of what men have been as a guide to what they are, he will give his attention to matters of very early times as well as to modern events. It is a matter of interest to know exact dates, and the names of principal figures, but history has a more important interest than that. The hows and whys of important movements and measures should be the particular objects of inquiry. Students very frequently give a great deal of attention to ancient and mediæval history, less frequently to more modern history. Commendable as this may be there is a history neglected in the schools that should be given a considerable part of the student's attention. I refer to current history. Let the student be directed to the daily doings of the world and it frees him from one form of narrow-mindedness. It teaches him to look upon the work of to-day as the important work, and to seriously consider the possibilities of the future. When the student is taught the use of books why should he not at the same time be taught the use of current periodicals? Is it not a great lesson to learn the distinction between the newspaper and the bitterly, or cunningly partizan political sheet? So to the old studies of ancient, mediæval, and modern history, let us add current history. It might not be out of place to mention just here that in historical study the student will come upon the frequent mention of physicians in important work that they have done not immediately connected with their profession. Such mention is, to say the least, a stimulus to the man who expects to follow in the same line of work.

It is supposed that in the study of the languages the student will be introduced to the choicest gems of their literatures. There is a wealth of worth in English and American literatures that need not be neglected. Does the medical student ask of this the old *cui bono?* Let Ruskin answer him. " We may, by good fortune, obtain a glimpse of a great poet, and hear the sound of his voice: or put a question to a man of science, and be answered good-humoredly. We may intrude ten minutes' talk on a cabinet minister, or snatch, once or twice in our lives, the privilege of throwing a bouquet on the path of a Princess, or arresting the kind glance of a Queen. And meantime there is a society continually open to us, of people who will talk to us as long as we like; talk to us in the best words we can choose; and this society, because it is so numerous and so gentle, and can be kept waiting round us all day long, not to grant audience, but to gain it, Kings and Statesmen lingering patiently in those plainly furnished and narrow ante-rooms, our book-case shelves, we make no account of that company, perhaps never listen to a word they would say all day long."

Another form of literature that should be included in the preliminary medical course is that created by the student. This is a form of work that should be made to come into almost every other form of work as a supplement. In the form of essays and arguments in writing the classes in history, language, and science can add to the interest and value of their work. It stimulates habits of careful thought and strengthens the memory. When original work of any kind is done, or when work is directed by an instructor in the laboratory, reports of the work should be required of each individual as it was done by him, the notes of the reports to have been made at the time the work was done. This is, in the egg, the noting, case-taking, and reporting of the careful physician. There should be in addition to this a special class for rhetoric, in which expression is properly taught. The usefulness of this will be apprecia-. ted by those who hope to add to the knowledge of the scientific world. The literary club should be fostered if excellence would be attained in this branch of work. It not only encourages essay work and the selection of good reading matter, but it also furnishes an opportunity for extemporaneous speaking which makes prompt thought necessary.

The preparatory medical course as arranged by a number of American schools includes a number of scientific studies of which biology is generally placed as the most important. Perhaps it is, but the spirit which originated the school preparatory to the study of medicine as we generally find it must have been a narrow one. There is one excuse for the school; it supplies what to some is a want, and without it there are those who would take something inferior, or nothing at all. It is a great deal better than nothing. The only preparatory school of medicine that should be encouraged should be the school that offers a general liberal education. The physician we wish to make is one who is symmetrical and is free from all tendencies towards parties or cliques. . He is a student of men and of affairs. Let him not then go, hermit-like, to any preparatory school except the school preparatory to living.

But there is so much that may be done; should a young man not select his studies, when it is possible, with some view to their future usefulness? This is altogether different from entering such a school as has been mentioned. Most schools permit some election of studies, and generally some of the Faculty will assist the student in making the wisest possible election, or when the work is done outside of a school the instructor or some capable friend will give the same assistance. The studies generally considered most useful to the student of medicine are the natural sciences. Of these what ones shall be chosen for careful attention? The answer should be as many as possible considering the time at the disposal of the student. Let it be kept in mind that there is such a dependence of the sciences each upon the other that not one can say of another, I have no need of thee. To do thorough work in natural science plenty of time must be given to it. Geology and mineralogy are of some special interest to the student of chemistry and materia medica, and if the student has the time at his disposal these studies should be given their full proportion of it. The only studies in natural science that will be spoken of particularly as having a special interest for the medical student are physics, chemistry, and the studies of life, or as it .is generally called, biology. These studies include also a number of special divisions that will be alluded to.

A number of the American medical colleges place physics in the list of studies for the matriculation examination. Physics has an importance that is not always recognized. The amount of ignorance that is sometimes displayed by medical students of such elementary physical forces as adhesion, elasticity and capillary attraction is something fearful and wonderful. The principal use of this branch of science to the medical man does not lie in its treatment of these forces. The medical student will wish to know something of the use of the microscope, and will naturally make a study of the eye and its conditions and diseases. Now is the time to make a beginning of each of these parts of his work by attention to the science of optics. Very rarely is much attention given in the medical schools to electricity and magnetism. Now is the time to prepare for the application of these forces to physiology, and to the treatment of disease. The art of taking a walk, depends, in a physical sense, upon certain forces that are treated of in the science of physics. There are more lessons in thinking in this work than the lesson in gravitation that a falling apple brought about. In the conduction of this study much more than class work should be attempted. The student should be given experiments to perform before the class, the apparatus of which should be made by himself. Laboratory work ought to be done in which the use of the more delicately made instruments is taught. There are works in the vicinity of every community that illustrate the practical application of a knowledge of physics to every day life. The student should be taught to visit these and to see with his brains as well as with his eyes. The exercise of reporting the extra-class and laboratory work has already been referred to. It can be used very advantageously in this study and in the two following.

Chemistry should come next in order. Chemistry is sometimes thought of as a medical study, but general chemistry certainly is not. General chemistry is in the course of almost every medical college, but it should be in the list of preliminary studies. Until the methods of teaching undergo very radical changes the majority of students will leave the medical colleges with a very imperfect knowledge of this science. Most students can make a rough analysis for albumen, and some can find glucose if it is present. I have seen a man who was called " Doctor " gravely look into it a vessel of urine and declare that there was no albumen there. Even among the better students chemistry is generally slighted, and can it be for any other reason than that there is generally not enough insight given to it to excite the student's interest? Within comparatively recent years laboratory work has been made a part of the medical course in chemistry and better work is being done than was before then. It is not necessary to speak of the importance of chemistry to the physician when it is already so recognized that re-agents are arranged in cases for bed-side use. I speak of this study among those of a man's preliminary education for more than one reason. It is one of the sciences that should be studied by everyone who wishes to have a liberal education. Its usefulness extends to every division of the world's work. It leads the way to a study of medical chemistry, and if medical chemistry alone was taught in the medical schools, as it should be, a knowledge of general chemistry would be necessary. In pursuing this study there are several things to be accomplished. With beginners the simpler laws of combination should first be studied. They should be illustrated by experiments so as to emphasize the laws and to familiarize the student with chemical apparatus and manipulation. This will lead the way to elementary laboratory work which should next be entered upon for the study of the more common elements. A beginning, too, should be made at this time in analysis. Before work in organic chemistry is begun the philosophy of chemistry should be studied. Organic chemistry is of particular importance to a physician for many important drugs and most of the dangerous poisons belong to this division. Much work can be done in organic chemistry both of learning what has already been done and of original work. Throughout the course, work in manufacturing chemistry and in analysis should be done in the laboratory. Complete as he may make such a course there will still be work in physiological chemistry and in the chemistry of medicines that may be done in the medical school.

In connection with the two sciences just spoken of there is a study which is valuable rather as an art than as a science to the physician. This is the photographic art. It is a duty which the painstaking physician owes to his profession to keep a record of his interesting cases. This art affords an opportunity to make a form of record that the pen cannot imitate. A bare allusion to photography is all that is allowable here, as it is not a study essential to the medical student, and if desirable the physician can study it with as much or more profit than the busy student.

The business of a physician is two-fold. He cares for people who are afflicted with disease, and he instructs those in health how they may avoid disease. How necessary it is then that he know what the conditions of health are. This knowledge is embraced in the studies of human anatomy and physiology and belongs to the medical course proper. In preparation for this let the student take a course of study in biology. He will, as a medical student, wish to know of prenatal life, of infancy and childhood, of manhood, and of old age—the development of the human being. All the world's a stage—in development, and the living beings are the players. Beginning as a cell the living thing goes on in its changes until it reaches adult life, when retrogressive changes commence, and finally, *sans* everything, it makes its exit. The student who is best prepared will see these same changes in everything. In adult form he sees the organism which attains perfection as a single cell. From this he is led to the higher forms of life in plants, and then through the various types of animal life. Again in embryology he sees a development from a single cell to a perfect animal that reminds him very much of the forms of life that he has seen in his earlier studies of perfect beings.

The course of study in biology should begin with work on general anatomy and physiology. It is best done in some such orderly manner as is suggested in the preceding paragraph. The simpler forms are best to start out with as they are seen even as a part of the higher organisms. It is important that the student be taught to collect his own specimens where this is possible, and to make his own preparations, both for temporary use and for preservation. The important work is in the laboratory where he is taught not only the facts that are known regarding his subjects, but also the use of instruments, and the best methods of study. The course in the laboratory should be continued through embryology and comparative anatomy. The work should teach the student familiarity with the microscope. He should learn to recognize the tissues as he sees them, and should know their origin and mode of growth. He should learn to inject his subjects for dissection and should acquire a knowledge of the use of the scalpel. The student who takes such a course as this is prepared for the study of human anatomy, the special points in histology, morbid anatomy, and the functions of the various organs of man—physiology.

Other branches of biology are studies of the individual characteristics of animals and plants. He who has a taste for such things will in some way find time for them. There is some value in the study of the habits and characteristics of animals, but if followed it is done most satisfactorily apart from school life. It affords rare advantanges for developing habits of observation, especially where the study is taken up naturally, and as a recreation rather than a regular employment.

In botany are most of the advantages that can be claimed for zoology. It has a practical advantage in the fact .that it leads directly to the study of medicinal plants. As generally studied, work is begun with the general structure and growth of plants, the peculiarities of plant life, and the variations in the anatomy and physiology of individuals. At this point plants are studied as individuals, and by the aid of a key the genus, species, and variety are. discovered. This method of study has some value to the medical student. It bears some analogy to the study of the symptoms of disease. It is, in fact, making a diagnosis. I believe, however, that the method can be improved upon. Let the old plan remain nearly as it has been, but add to it other exercises. The specimens instead of being furnished by the instructor, should be gathered by the student, and specimens of the same plant from seed to "old age" should be collected for study. This affords the student the benefit of out-of-door life, and gives him a practical knowledge of the plant that is not always obtained. He learns in this way the time of year of flowering, and seeding; the soil best suited to its growth ; and what other plants it has for near neighbors. The plant should be studied first without an artificial key. Each part should be taken up one at a time and its special peculiarities carefully noted. Groups should be made so familiar that a key would not be necessary for their recognition. The microscope should be used diligently in this work.

In each branch of biological study the student should be required to make drawings of his preparations,—not for the artistic value of the drawings, but because the practice calls attention to the forms of the parts and to the details of their structure. The drawing of microscopic specimens should also be required.

In this plan of a preliminary education I would give to music, and to drawing and painting a more prominent part than they are generally made to play. They are regarded too much in the light of luxuries, whereas they have not a little value as educators. Some attention is given to vocal music and to drawing in almost all schools, but I would have them consume a considerably greater part of the student's attention than can be done in these studies as the school courses are arranged. More thorough work can be done out of school, and the work can more easily be made to take the place of recreation. These branches of study have a refining influence over a person's life, and would be worth cultivating for that alone. To the student and physician they have a special value. One study developes the sense of hearing and the other the sense of sight. In these days when so much attention is given to examination for color-blindness and for acuteness of hearing it behooves the physician to be himself as nearly perfect as possible. If the student will practice upon some musical instrument, as I believe would be better for him, whether it be piano, flute, or violin, he will acquire a use of his fingers that he will one day be thankful for. As ophthalmologist, surgeon, obstetrician, gynecologist,—what branch of the medical profession does not require the use of nimble fingers, and a delicate, gentle, certain touch ? To him who has eyes and will see, music will show a valuable moral lesson. The student makes no objection to the constant practice of exercises in music that have for their object the development of easy and rapid movements—the discipline of the hand. Will he then object to mental occupation simply because the opprobrious title *disciplinary* can be applied to it?

In drawing and painting there are uses that the student of medicine should not ignore. They will teach the observance of apparent trifles,—a point in education that is well worth noting. They teach the observance of variations in shade and color. They teach one to look not only for usual appearances, but for the unexpected. They are valuable as serving to hold the attention and to quicken the memory if used in connection with other studies. Let dissections be copied in crayon or colors, and the arrangement of apparatus be drawn in connection with laboratory work, and the student will have accomplished much more than in the simple performance of the work.

There is certain work that a person expecting to study medicine ought to know something about, but which does not belong to general school work, nor properly to the medical course. There may be several of these studies (they may be called studies in this connection), but there are two to which I would especially call attention.

The first is the art of cooking. Does it cause a smile ? Look at it soberly. Bad cooking is the cause of a large percentage of bad health. The most valuable work of a physician is prophylactic. The natural inference is that a physician to be fully prepared for work should know something of the proper methods of cooking. A student with this knowledge will better appreciate certain parts of his medical course,—particularly hygiene, physiology, and the practice of medicine. There is a right way and a wrong way to cook. The right way, it is hardly necessary to say, is the one to learn. If one could also learn a little of the methods of bad cooks, it would be an advantage from a medical stand-point. The proper place to learn the art is in the kitchen under the direction of a good cook. This subject will direct the student's attention to the kindred subject of diet,—of proper food, as well as the proper preparation of it.

The second of the studies spoken of is practical nursing. At first thought it might seem that this belonged to the medical course—but does it? There are very few medical students who leave the college with any experience in nursing, and after receiving the degree it is almost impossible to gain any, such experience. The college might introduce it in connection with its clinical work, but at the clinics the patients who receive treatment, as a rule, do not require the services of a professional nurse, and even if they did and the students supplied the demand, their work as nurses would interfere with their college work. Or the preceptor might install his student as nurse in those cases in which there was peculiar interest. But even here it is not only often inconvenient for student and patient, but it also interferes with the study hours of the student. Besides the convenience there is another reason for preferring that experience in nursing should be had before beginning medical student life. Nursing is the link of separation between professional medical work and secular work. It is a more practical preparation for the study of the scientific management of disease than any other one study that can be mentioned. The odd times of leisure can be used in rendering assistance to neighbors and acquaintances who have sickness in their families. There are many valuable lessons to be learned by an acting nurse. One is the value of golden silence. There are many questions that should never be asked, and more that should never be answered. Other lessons are obedience to an authority, the care of the sick room, and the thousand little things that must be done for the comfort of the patient.

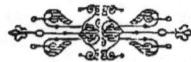

PART III.

A COLLEGE COURSE OF STUDY.

By most students a systematic course of study is
desired. It has already been stated that as a rule a better
education is obtained in a school than out of it. The
purpose of Part III is to suggest a selection of studies for
the young man who carries·his educational work through a
college of the liberal arts.

It might be well to begin by stating what requirements
should be made for entrance to the course to be suggested.
It is arranged for an American student at an American
college.

English :

English Grammar, with Analysis.

English Composition. An essay to be written at the
time and place of examination upon a subject announced
by the examiners.

Spelling and Penmanship. To be criticised from a dictation exercise, and from the general examination papers.

Some familiarity with the best English and American writers.

Geography:

Elements of Physical Geography.

Political Geography, with special reference to the United States.

The study and examination in Ancient Geography to be in connection with the work in Ancient Languages.

History:

Outlines of General History.

History of the United States.

Ancient History of Rome and Greece in connection with the work in Greek and Latin.

Some familiarity with the principal current events of the world.

Mathematics:

Arithmetic. including the Metric System.

Algebra, through Quadratic Equations.

Geometry, Plane and Solid.

Plane Trigonometry.

German and French:

German preferred if but one is offered. Easy reading, and some knowledge of pronunciation and grammar. The student to be ranked A, if both are offered; B 1, if German only; and B 2, if French only is offered.

Latin:

Grammar, including Prosody.

Cæsar, Gallic War, four books.

Sallust, Cataline, or Jugurthine War.

Cicero, five orations.

Virgil, Æneid, six books.

Latin Prose Composition, construction of simple sentences.

Greek:

Grammar, including Prosody.

Xenophon, Anabasis, four books.

Homer, Iliad, three books.

Greek Prose Composition, construction of simple sentences.

Elementary Physics.

These are much more than the requirements for entrance to any of the American medical colleges, but are less than most of the brighter students are willing to be satisfied with. If the course is pursued as all student work should be, the student should be prepared to enter any of the American colleges of the liberal arts. The following is recommended as a college course for one desirous of preparing for the study of medicine. It may be pursued in any or the American colleges with the exception of a few low-grade colleges where the course is hardly equivalent to the course in a good academy. Authors are not given as the work of colleges differs widely, especially as regards the work in Latin and Greek, and what is desired is a certain method and quality of work.

44

Latin Language and Literature.   Latin Prose Composition.
Greek Language and Literature.   Greek Prose Composition.
In connection with these two, the study of Antiquities, Geography, and History.
:   Mathematics,—Spherical Trigonometry, and Analytical Geometry.
Botany.
English Composition, and Declamations.

Latin and Greek continued from the Freshman Year.
Mathematics,—Calculus, and Mechanics.
Physics.   Special work in Physics, with Laboratory Exercises.
English Composition, and Declamations.

German or French.   Under certain circumstances both may be studied.
Chemistry, with Laboratory Exercises.
English History.
English Literature.
Logic.
Psychology.
English Composition.   Orations.

SENIOR YEAR.

German, or French, continued from the Junior Year.
Biology, with Laboratory Exercises.
Ethics.
American History.
American Literature.
Theory of Government.
Sanitary, and Social Science.
English Composition.   Orations.

Throughout the course of four years there should be a weekly exercise reviewing the current history of the world, in which attention should be directed to general political affairs, and to such other matters as are of general interest.

There should also be a course in drawing.   In certain cases coloring should be taught.

This course, it will be observed, is chiefly designed for the purpose of discipline.   *Discipline* is to many a harsh word; would it sound any better if I said—for the purpose of development?   As has been suggested before there is no general educational course suitable only for the student who intends presently to study medicine.   Discipline is the German watchword.   It is by means of their very thorough discipline that the German students have cultivated their love for research for its own sake.   There are certain of the studies that have been placed in the course because of their usefulness to the student in his future work, certain others because they start, as a fountain, the channel of his thoughts towards what he regards as an important part of his life-work, and others again because they prepare him to live as a man among men.

www.ingramcontent.com/pod-product-compliance
Lightning Source LLC
Chambersburg PA
CBHW022029190326
41519CB00010B/1639